MY POSITIVE UNCLE

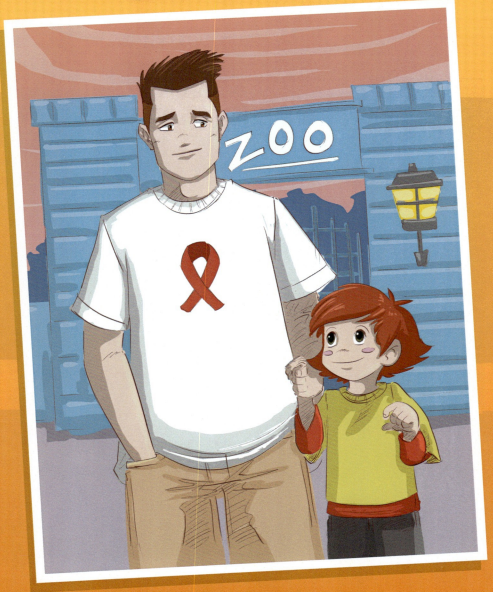

Dr. Wallace Wong

To order additional copies of this book, contact:
Xlibris
1-888-795-4274
www.Xlibris.com
Orders@Xlibris.com

Illustrated by Salvador Capuyan

ISBN: Softcover   978-1-7960-5160-5
        EBook   978-1-7960-5159-9

Print information available on the last page

Rev. date: 10/31/2019

MY POSITIVE UNCLE

Dr. Wallace Wong

Illustrated by
Salvador Capuyan

INTRODUCTION

HIV does not just affect individuals living with HIV. It also affects their family and loved ones— especially children. Children tend to be relatively concrete in their thinking, thus they may not be able to understand the complexity of the health issue.

With the advanced treatments that are now available, people living with HIV can live long and healthy lives. Since people living with HIV are living longer, the overall number of this population will increase. Unfortunately, many parents or family members living with HIV often find it difficult to talk to younger family members (e.g. children) about HIV. This air of discomfort can create anxiety in the child and cause tension within the family. Many fear that children may tell others, which in turn may cause the child to be stigmatized and ostracized. Further, parents or family members living with HIV may find it difficult to share affection with their children, fearing that they may be contagious and infect the children, despite evidence to the contrary.

Children in various developmental stages need to build attachment through sharing affection with their parents and family members. Without such affection, strong bonds within the family may be lost and leave the child feeling disconnected.

My Positive Uncle is a children's book written in simple language. I hope it will help bridge the gap for parents or other family members to open up the dialogue about this important issue. I believe that open communication is important to help clarify unnecessary myths and fear that exists surrounding this health issue.

FOREWORD

This book is written for children learning more about people living with HIV and demystifying common misconceptions about people living with HIV. This book is suitable for children from grades 3 and up. Parents are encouraged to use this book to talk with children younger than grade 3 as long as they modify the language and content to fit the child's developmental level and understanding. Open and ongoing communication will be the best way to address different sensitive issues addressed in this book.

One of the most common ways to transfer the HIV virus is through unprotected sexual activities. This book does not go into detail about this subject. I would like to leave it to the parents or caretakers to decide when is an appropriate time to address this piece. Of course, early education and discussion is always better, as it helps the child to understand that it is safe to talk about this and other topics, and it is safe to ask questions. Most of all, education enhances protection and safety. Different research suggests that children and youth who have had sexual health education tend to have fewer unplanned pregnancies and fewer sexually transmitted diseases.

Like any sexual related education, it is often challenging for parents to discuss these topics with their children. Often times it is easier to talk about these topics with other people or even other people's children, except for your own. I hope this book will serve a small part in opening up the conversation about this subject. Whether we like to admit it or not, our children are exposed to and are thinking about different sexual related topics. It is important to be a good role model for your children and to openly discuss these topics.

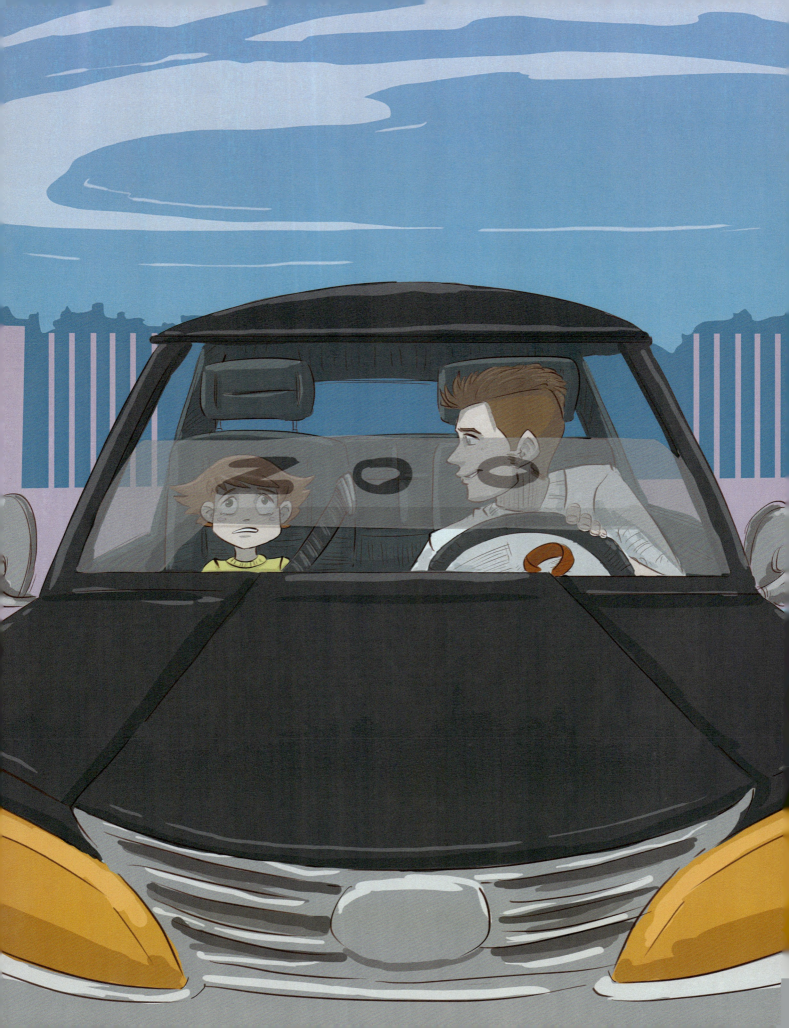

CHAPTER 1

Tyler is sitting in the car with his Uncle Joe. They are going to the zoo today. Tyler is very excited because he is going to see many different animals and is able to spend time with his favorite uncle. Tyler has not seen Uncle Joe for several months. The last time was when Uncle Joe came to visit Tyler and his mother, sharing with them that he was HIV positive. Tyler heard about people living with HIV before and different people seem to have different opinions about this. Some say it is contagious and some say it is a very deadly virus.

Tyler knows very little about it and he really wants to learn more of the facts about people living with HIV because he cares a lot about his Uncle Joe.

Tyler has so many questions but he does not know where to begin and does not know how to ask questions without upsetting Uncle Joe.

Uncle Joe senses Tyler's uneasiness so he says, "Tyler, I know you have many questions about my health and I'd love to answer any questions that you have."

Tyler feels a sense of relief and replies, "Thank you Uncle Joe. I'll let you know if I think of any questions."

When they finally arrive at the zoo, Tyler can hardly wait to get out of the car. He is full of excitement, waiting to spend a day with Uncle Joe and see different animals in the zoo.

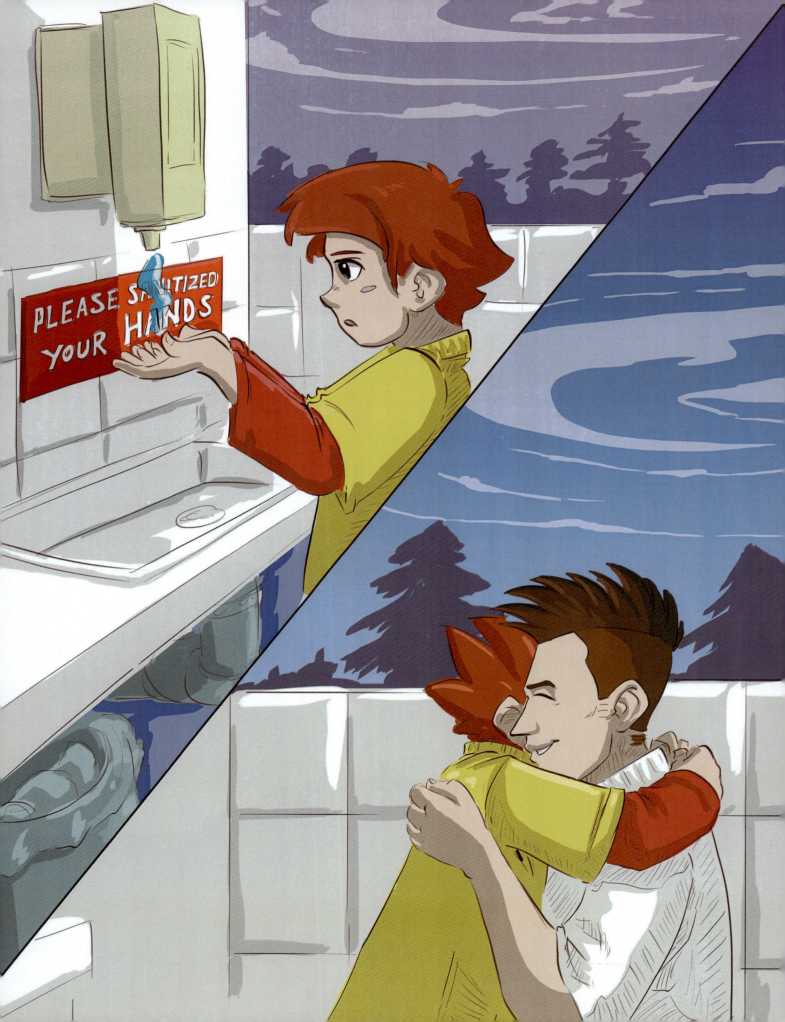

Chapter 2

Uncle Joe purchases the tickets and they walk inside the zoo's gate. Tyler sees a sign that says "Please sanitize your hands". He then thinks of a question to ask Uncle Joe.

He looks at Uncle Joe and asks, "Uncle Joe, is it safe to hug or hold hands with people who are living with HIV?"

Uncle Joe smiles as he is pleased that Tyler feels comfortable asking the question. He replies, "HIV is a very tiny organism that can only live in our blood stream or bodily fluids. It can't survive outside of the body so you won't get HIV from touching someone, hugging them or shaking their hand. You don't get HIV through casual contact*. So, if you like, you can hold my hand or you can give me a hug and not have to worry about getting the virus**."

Tyler happily throws Uncle Joe a big hug because he has really misses seeing him.

Tyler then asks, "Uncle Joe, how does the HIV virus pass to other people?"

Uncle Joe kneels down and says, "That is a very good question. HIV can only be passed on to another person through infected bodily fluids, such as blood, semen****, and breast milk, and these bodily fluids need to get into another person's bloodstream."

Tyler expresses bewilderment about what he is learning and wants to ask more questions. Uncle Joe reassures him, "Don't worry, I will explain more to you later. We have a whole day to spend together."

---

* Casual contact: Casual contact includes touching, hugging, hand shaking and social kissing. These levels of contact do not cause a person to be infected by this communicable disease from another infected person.

** Virus: A very tiny collective of organic matter that is able to self-replicate and is capable of infecting a cell, which may cause disease. However, Viruses lack the capacity to live out of a host body.

*** Semen: is a white bodily fluid that is secreted by the gonads of male animals. It carries sperm that helps facilitate fertilization of the female animals.

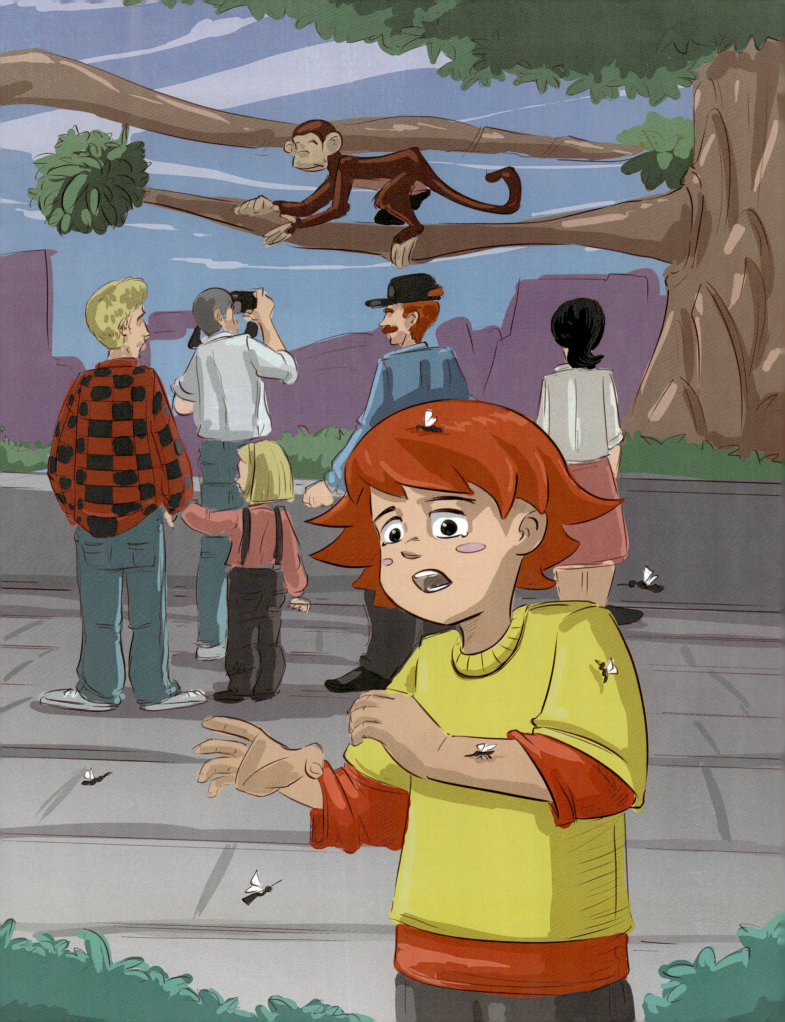

Chapter 3

Tyler really wants to see the monkeys at the Monkey Jungle Exhibit. When they get there, Tyler sees many monkeys. Some are sleeping, some are swinging on tree branches, and some young monkeys are sitting by their mothers.

Tyler loves this exhibit, but he also notices that there are many mosquitos flying around this place. Very soon, he finds a few mosquito bites on both Uncle Joe's and his own legs. Tyler remembers that mosquitos love sucking people's blood. The same mosquito could have bitten Uncle Joe and then bit him. He wonders if this will pass the HIV virus onto him.

Tyler asks Uncle Joe in a hurry, "Uncle Joe, can I get HIV from a mosquito bite if the same mosquito bites you and I?"

Uncle Joe smiles and says, "No, you do not get the HIV virus from a mosquito bite. When a mosquito bites me and sucks my blood, the mosquito does not re-inject the blood into the new person. Since there is no blood transmission* from the mosquito, it is not possible for the HIV virus to pass to another person." Uncle Joe continues, "Mosquitoes are known to carry different infectious diseases; including malaria and yellow fever— but HIV is not one of them. There are millions of mosquitos in this world. If their bites could pass the HIV virus, many people would have been affected."

Uncle Joe reaches into his bag and puts some mosquito repellent on Tyler. Tyler feels happy that he asked Uncle Joe this question. He feels less worried about this now.

---

* Blood transmission: Blood transmission is to transfer blood or blood products from one person to another person

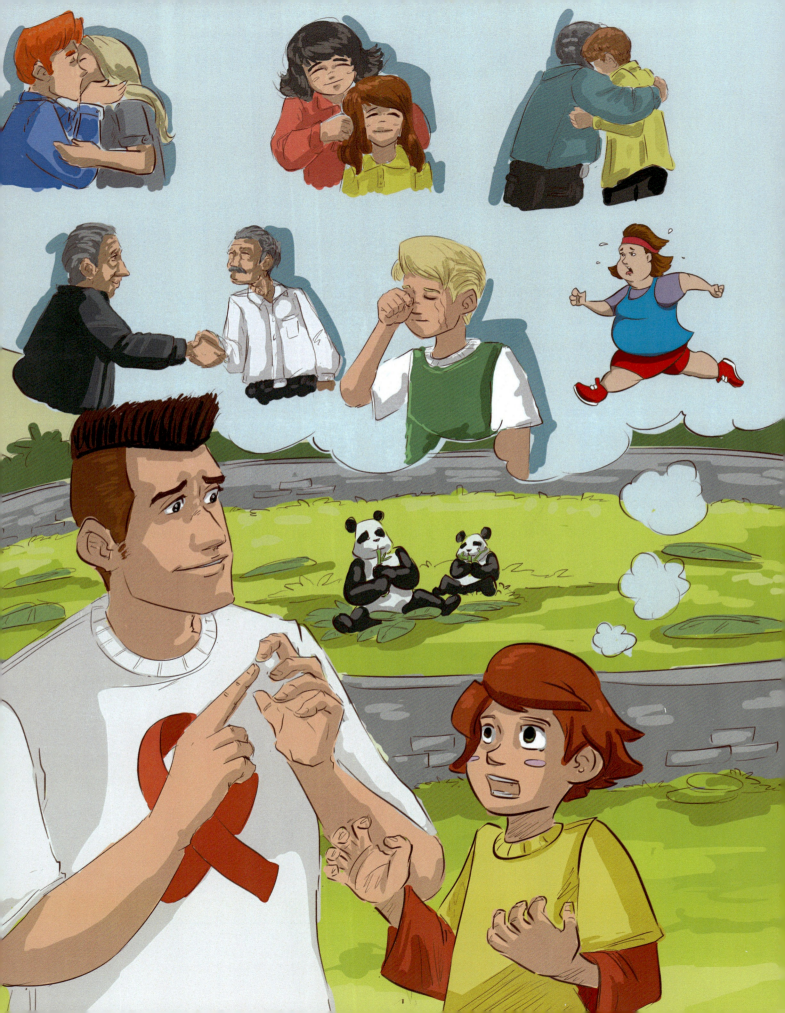

CHAPTER 4

After the Monkey Jungle Exhibit, Tyler wants to see the panda. The zoo is quite big and they are walking under the sun. Soon, they are both sweating from the heat. Tyler can feel his Uncle's hand is sweating from holding his hand. Tyler remembers Uncle Joe said that the HIV virus can only pass through bodily fluids. He knows the chance for the HIV virus to pass through sweat is unlikely, but he thinks it will be important to know all the facts. Tyler looks up to Uncle Joe and asks, "Can someone get the HIV virus by touching the sweat of people living with HIV?"

Uncle Joe replies, "No. You do not get HIV by casual touching, such as hugging or kissing someone living with HIV. HIV cannot be transmitted through sweat, tears, urine, or saliva. That's another great question, Tyler!"

"So you can kiss me and it is okay?" Tyler asks excitedly. Uncle Joe nods his head.

"Of course it is." Uncle Joe then gives Tyler a big kiss on his cheek and Tyler feels so happy and so close to his uncle again.

"How about brushing their hair?" Tyler is trying to check further into this. Uncles Joe shakes his head.

"How about shaking their hands?" Tyler is now trying to be cheeky. Uncle Joe begins to laugh and says, "No dear. It's perfectly safe."

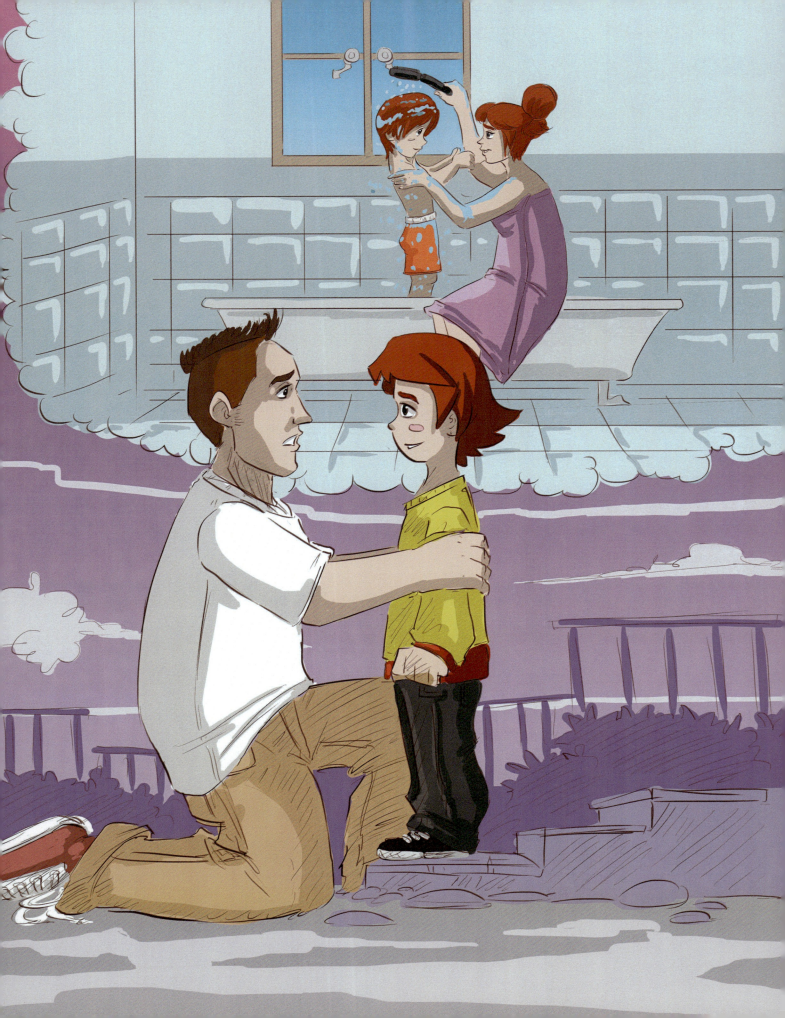

CHAPTER 5

When they arrive at the panda exhibit, there are many children observing the panda and they are just as excited as Tyler.

Tyler finds a good spot to see the mother panda bathing the baby panda. They seem be to having a great time. Tyler tries to be smart and say, "Uncle Joe, let me tell you this. A person will not get HIV from sharing the same bath with another person living with HIV!"

Uncle Joe laughs, "It's very true, but can you tell me why that is the case?"

Tyler thinks for a moment, "Well, there is no exchange of bodily fluids, and bathing together is casual contact. So, it is not possible for someone to get HIV from bathing together or sharing the bathwater."

Uncle Joe replies, "That's right. In fact, you won't get HIV through sharing soap, bath water, or towels."

While Tyler is feeling proud of his answer, he realizes that he feels hungry. It's already lunch time.

Tyler asks, "I am hungry Uncle Joe. Can we have lunch?"

Uncle Joe pats Tyler's head, "Of course! I am hungry too."

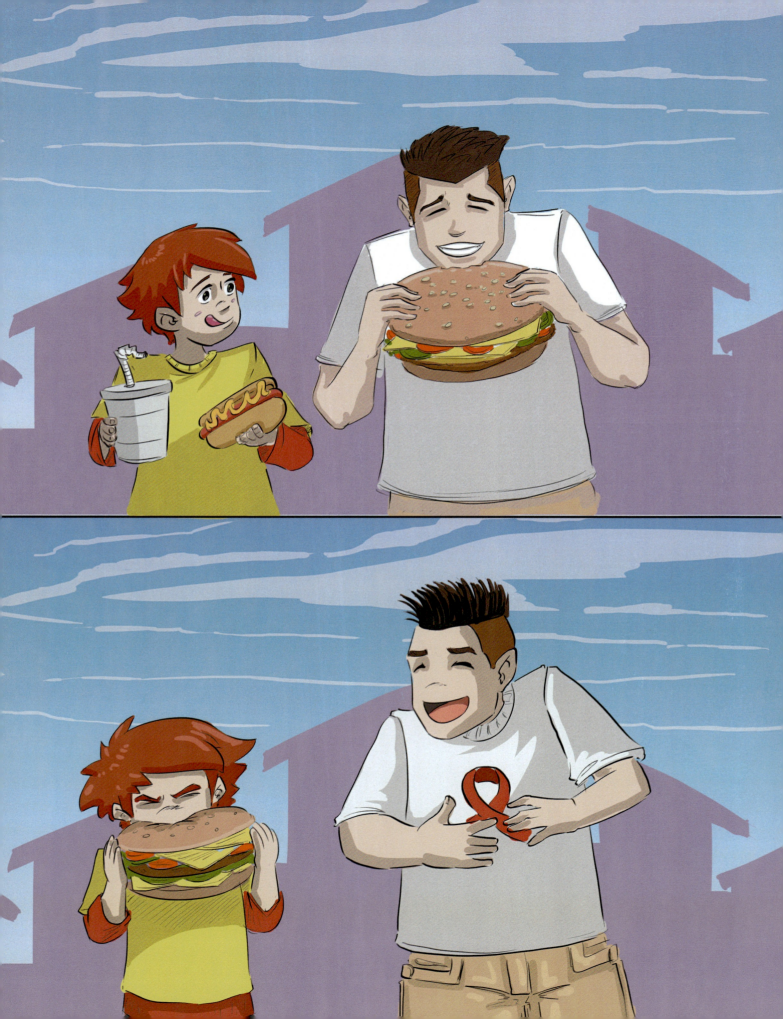

Chapter 6

The zoo's cafeteria is located on the top of a small hill. Tyler can see the entire city outside of the cafeteria.

Tyler decides that he wants a hot dog and Uncle Joe says he will have a cheeseburger.

Tyler really enjoys looking at the view while eating his hot dog, but he can't help noticing how delicious Uncle Joe's cheeseburger looks. He keeps watching Uncle Joe taking big bites of his burger.

Tyler was just about to ask Uncle Joe for a bite of his cheeseburger, but he remembers his mother warned him about sharing food, because germs can be transmitted from one person to another through food sharing.

Uncle Joe also notices Tyler looking at his cheeseburger. He offers Tyler a bite. Tyler looks hesitant and says, "Will I get HIV if I share your food?"

"Good question." Uncle Joe says, "HIV is not bacteria. Remember earlier we learned that HIV is a virus, which is different than bacteria. A virus cannot live outside the body, so a person living with HIV can cook and share meals with anyone without passing the virus to anyone else. A person living with HIV can cook and share utensils with you without passing the HIV virus to you. You won't get infected from sharing meals or drinks either."

"Yeah!" Tyler cheers, "Now can I have a bite of your burger?"

Tyler takes a big bite of the burger and he loves it.

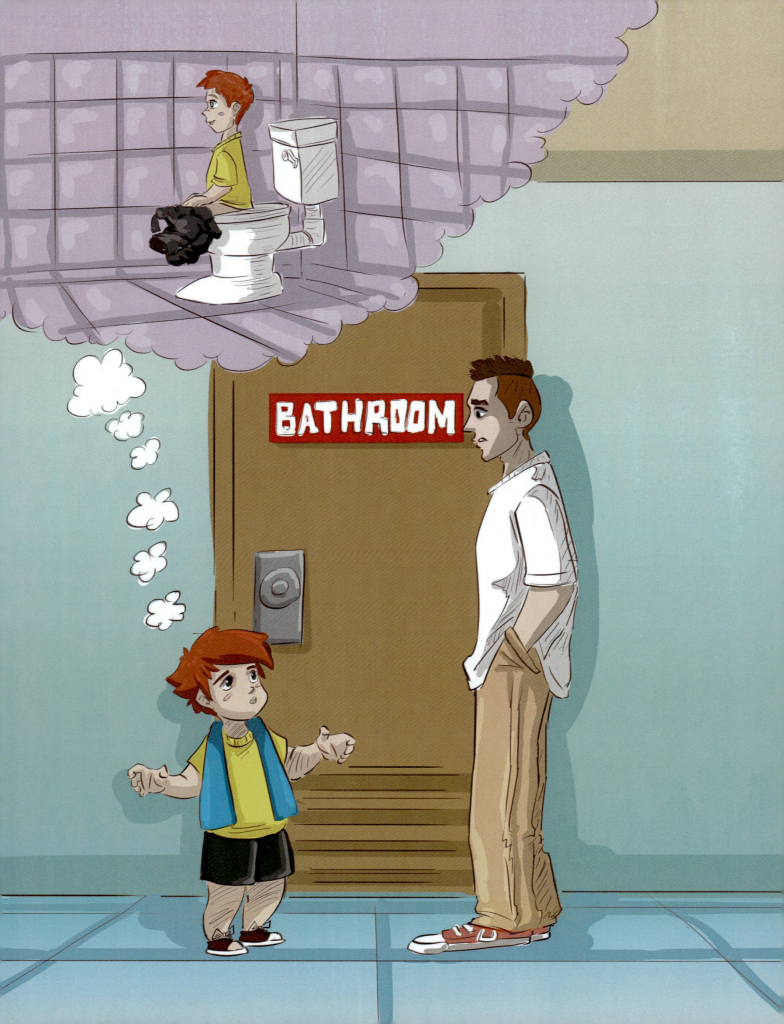

BATHROOM

CHAPTER 7

After the delicious lunch, they go to see the polar bears, elephants, tigers, and wolves.

Tyler is fascinated by all the animals.

He realizes that he has not been to the bathroom for a long time and now he has to go.

As Uncle Joe walks him to the bathroom, Tyler proudly says to Uncle Joe, "I bet a person cannot get HIV through sharing toilet seats."

Uncle Joe can't help laughing, "Yes, you are getting very smart. But do you know why?"

"Well, there is no exchange of bodily fluid and sharing a toilet seat is a casual contact, so it is not possible to pass on HIV through sharing toilet seats."

"Very true. Did you know that HIV can't survive on surfaces? That means you can't get HIV through sharing things with a person living with HIV."

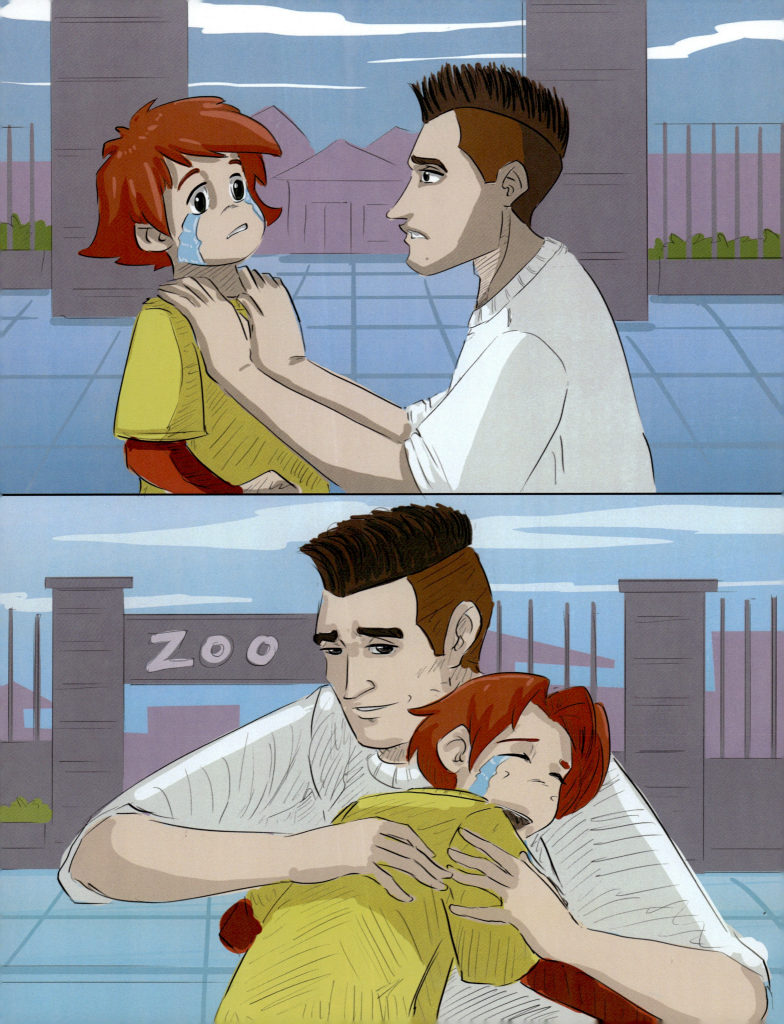

CHAPTER 8

After a long and fun day, Tyler can't recall all of the animals that he saw but he knows that he will always remember this special day that he spent with his Uncle Joe.

Even though Tyler asked Uncle Joe a lot of questions, he still has a big question that he wanted to ask all day. He was afraid to ask the question in case the answer is not what he wants to hear.

Uncle Joe notices Tyler looking nervous. "Tyler, what's wrong? Didn't you have a good day today?"

Tyler nods and gives Uncle Joe a big hug.

"What's wrong, Tyler?"

Tyler cannot hold this question in any longer and his eyes begin to get teary, "Uncle Joe, are you going to die soon because you are living with HIV? I heard people die from this."

Uncle Joe looks into Tyler's eyes and says, "No, I will not die soon just because I am living with HIV. HIV is no longer a terminal illness, especially with the advancement of current medicine. My medication helps keep the HIV virus under control. As long as I take the medication and live a healthy lifestyle, I will stay healthy for a long time."

Tyler felt so relieved when he heard this, and said, "I love you Uncle Joe and I don't want you to go anywhere."

"Don't worry Tyler, I will be around for a long time and spend many more fun days with you."

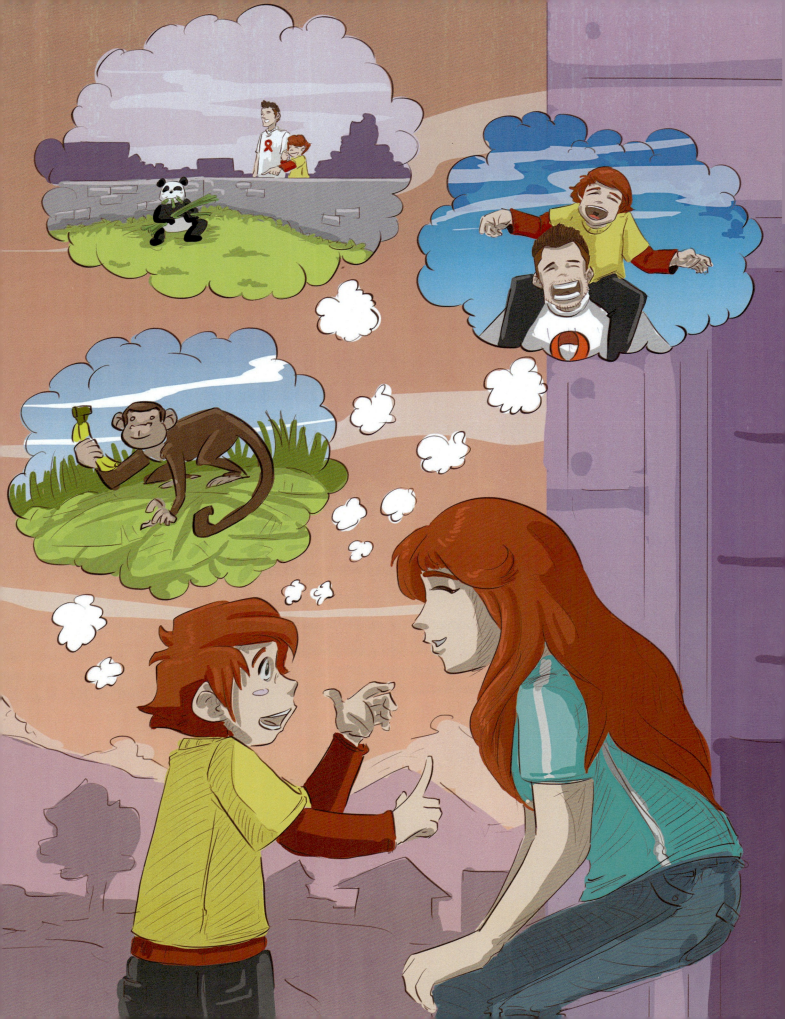

CHAPTER 9

When Tyler gets home, he rushes to tell his mom about his day and the conversations he had with Uncle Joe. Tyler's mother is so happy that he had a fun time with Uncle Joe and that he had a chance to talk to Uncle Joe about the questions that had been bothering him for some time.

Tyler felt glad that he got to spend the day with Uncle Joe.

He also felt proud that he asked those questions, because he would have kept feeling confused and worried if he did not know the answers.

He realizes that he has learned a lot today. He has also learned how much he loves his Uncle Joe and how much he wants to spend more time with him. In fact, Tyler is already thinking about where he and Uncle Joe will go next.

The End

Printed in the United States
By Bookmasters